Situation BMA
Judgement
Test

D1350106

How to approach the test
with mock questions,
answers and full
explanations

DR ALEX AL-SHAIKH

DR DARRAGH HODNETT

Ordering Information:Quantity sales. Special discounts are available on quantity purchases by corporations, associations, and others. For details, contact the publisher at the address above. Orders by UK trade bookstores and wholesalers.

Please contact Simon Cowen Publishing Or visit scowenpublishing.com

All content is owned by the authors and official information regarding the test is taken from the official site www.foundationprogramme.nhs.uk

The information within this resource is intended solely as a revision aid for the Situation Judgment Test . Any information within this book is produced by the authors and are only their opinions. The material presented is for individual private-study only; public performance of the material without written permission is specifically forbidden. All the learning resources are copyright. The views expressed are those of the authors and not those of any sponsors or partners.

Publisher's Cataloging-in-Publication data

Copyright © 2014 by Simon Cowen Publishing

ISBN-13: 978-0990853817
ISBN-10: 0990853810

What is the SJT?

The Situational Judgement Test (SJT) is an examination undertaken by all those wishing to enter the foundation programme in the United Kingdom. The examination itself consists of 70 questions, which must be completed within 2 hours and 20 minutes leaving 2 minutes per question.

The examination contains two different types of question; ranking questions where the candidate must rank a series of 5 responses to a given scenario in order of most to least appropriate and multiple response questions where the candidate must select the three most appropriate responses to a given scenario out of a choice of seven.

The SJT is a particularly important examination for final year medically students as it comprises 50% of the total score used to select which foundation school a candidate is allocated to. The other 50% is made up from the candidate's performance to date at medical school (educational performance measure (EPM)) as well as other academic achievements such as additional degrees or publications. However, it can be argued that the SJT is even more important than the EPM. This is because one can score anywhere from 0-50 on the SJT however the minimum one can score on their EPM is 34 meaning that there is further to fall if a candidate does not do well on the SJT compared to their EPM. It is therefore vital to

3

score well on the SJT if a candidate wants to be allocated to a competitive foundation school.

SJTs are now used in the selection process for a number of different careers not just medicine. The aim of the test is to see how a candidate responds to different potentially challenging situations in the workplace.

The candidate's responses are then compared to a "model answer" which has been developed by a panel of experts who decide what the most appropriate response would be to each situation.

This has a number of advantages over previously used systems to allocate candidates to foundation programme places. Not least it removes any bias by undertaking the test in invigilated exam conditions. It has also been shown to have a reduced level of impact from other non-modifiable factors such as gender and ethnicity. The scenarios presented in the SJT are all scenarios that it is entirely possible an FY1 doctor could face when working. It therefore has a good level of validity although as the test has only been running for 2 years previously it is yet to be seen whether those who score well on the SJT become more competent doctors.

Key Themes when Answering Questions

When answering SJT questions it is important to remember that the appropriate response is what an FY1 doctor should do, not what you would do. With this in mind it is important to approach each question with some important basic rules and also to understand the guidance given to all doctors by the GMC in their "Good Medical Practice" document which is available both online and in paper form. It is highly recommended that candidates read this document prior to sitting the SJT.

The document is split into four key domains; 1) knowledge, skills and performance, 2) safety and quality, 3) communication, partnership and teamwork and 4) maintaining trust.

The first domain deals with the importance of developing and maintaining a good standard of performance by keeping up to date with the latest guidelines as well as new developments in research. It also deals with the importance of the concept of medicine being a career with lifelong learning and that this learning should be applied to a doctor's everyday practice. This domain also states the importance of proper documentation which is both accurate as well as clear in order for patient care to be continuous and efficient.

The second domain deals with the importance of cooperating with and contributing to safety nets put in place to protect patients. It also deals with the importance of responding appropriately when patient safety may be at risk either through factors under your personal control or those where appropriate escalation is required.

The third domain discusses the importance of effective communication both with colleagues as well as patients. This should also include an implication that doctors should contribute to the training as well as the support of students as well as junior doctors attached to their teams. However, this must not impact on patient care. This domain also highlights the importance of effective communication when handing patients over between care providers.

The final domain deals with the importance of maintaining trust both on a doctor patient level as well as maintaining trust in the medical profession as a whole. It highlights the importance of treating both patients and colleagues without discrimination as well as acting with honesty and integrity at all times. This includes non-clinical areas such as when asked for legal opinions or when dealing with financial matters where potential conflicts of interest may arise.

Time Constraints and Practicalities of the Exam

As previously detailed, the SJT exam is a fast-paced exam. There is generally quite a lot of text to read for each question and it is vital to spend no more than 2 minutes per question in order to finish in the allocated time. As there is no negative marking, there is no benefit to leaving questions blank if you are unsure or if you do not have time to complete the test.

A candidate who leaves the answer blank for a "ranking" style question will gain 0/20 marks, whereas a candidate who fills in answers (even if completely incorrectly) will gain 8/20 marks. Therefore, it is better to "guess" in order to complete the exam if you are running low on time.

An unfortunate pitfall for some candidates is to answer the questions on the question paper then attempt to fill in the answers onto the answer sheet at the end of the examination- this increases the risk of not finishing in time and the error rate of transferring answers across can lead to problems for some candidates.

It is important to be aware of the format of the answer sheet that is used in the SJT. It is relatively complex if you have not used a similar sheet before. An example of the answer sheet is widely available online.

Narrowing your choices

It is usually possible to ease the task of choosing the correct responses in both formats of questions. In the ranking questions there is usually one response that will appear completely inappropriate, and thus you are able to rank this bottom. Likewise with the selection questions ("choose the three best responses) there will be a couple of responses of the eight possibilities that are obviously incorrect.

It may be useful to cross these off and leave yourself with a smaller pool of answers to choose the potential three correct answers from.

Determining the exact question

It is vital to read the question carefully to ascertain what exactly is being asked. The questions will be specifically worded in such a fashion as to make it clear what the thrust of the question is. For example, some questions will ask for the "initial" three responses you would carry out. This indicates that long drawn out processes such as filling in clinical incident forms or informing clinical supervisors are not the correct answers despite potentially being good clinical practice and good courses of action in the longer term. In these sort of questions answers that relate acutely to patient safety will be more likely to be correct, eg. "go and assess the patient".

It is also important to be clear in the differences between ranking style questions and questions which ask you to choose the 3 best responses. Examples of both are given in this book and the different approaches that are required for each type are also explained. In the ranking questions there is usually one response that will appear completely inappropriate, and thus you are able to rank this bottom. Likewise with the selection questions there will be a couple of responses that are obviously incorrect. It may be useful to cross these off and leave yourself with a smaller pool of answers to choose the potential three correct answers from.

General approach

Whilst it is impossible to create a list of "rules" to follow to be able to answer all SJT questions, there is a general approach that can help rank responses to the majority of questions. There are only a limited number of themes that run throughout SJT questions.

Patient safety- This is of utmost importance and only answers that preserve patient safety are acceptable. This can make it straightforward to rule out certain responses. A good idea may be to approach each response with the simple thought; "does this potentially endanger patient safety?"

A particular theme of the SJT is the fact that you should question senior decision making if you feel it will harm patient safety- however uncomfortable this may be for yourself or your seniors. For example if a senior doctor has decided to discharge a patient but you review the patient later and feel this is not correct it is entirely within reason to act in the best interests of the patient as you see fit.

Probity- This is extremely important in the public perception of a good doctor, and is also frequently highlighted by the GMC. Second to patient safety this is the most important consideration, so if a response to a question involves dishonesty in any fashion this will be an inappropriate response.

Knowing the limits of you practice- It would be regarded as unsafe to perform any task above that normally expected of an F1. This includes unsupervised practical procedures such as chest drains/ lumbar punctures, discharging of patients and outpatient prescriptions. It is also not usually expected for an F1 to break bad news to a patient unless no other doctor is available to do so. Additionally, it is inappropriate for a doctor to consent a patient for a procedure they are themselves unable to carry out. These are simple rules, but are helpful in identifying unsafe and inappropriate answers to some SJT questions.

Responsibility- It is important to take responsibility for you actions. For example if you sign in a drug chart, you are responsible for the prescription even if a senior has told you to do so. Therefore you must satisfy yourself that you are happy that you are making safe decisions. Another theme of the SJT is the fact that you should question senior decision making if you feel it will harm patient safety- however uncomfortable this may be for yourself or your seniors. For example if a senior doctor has decided to discharge a patient but you review the patient later and feel this is not correct it is entirely within reason to act in the best interests of the patient as you see fit.

Reporting- In general in SJT questions it is advisable to prioritise acting in the immediate term and reporting later. When you are required to report or inform a senior of a situation it is usually best to inform your direct senior (as an Fɪ this would be an SHO) if given an option rather than going straight to very senior people such as your consultant, the GMC or the Foundation Director. However if the situation was acutely very serious or a patient was acutely unwell it may be appropriate to skip some levels of seniority or even go straight to the consultant responsible for the patient. If you need to report something to people who is not directly responsible for the patient or there is a question of a colleagues' probity a clinical incident form or the foundation director may be more appropriate.

Work-life balance- This is an important theme that runs throughout the SJT questions. It is regarded that a good work-life balance is vital to ensure the highest standards of practice when you are in the hospital. This means that it is not good practice to be staying late every day or going back into the hospital if you realise that you have forgotten to do something. The exception to this is when patient safety is potentially compromised- although there are often other options that maintain patient safety such as handing over to the oncall team which would be appropriate responses.

Colleague relationships- The SJT contains many questions that involve colleague relationships. It is advisable to choose empathic responses to these questions; gently attempting to elucidate the cause of a problem is better than confronting your colleague or ignoring the issue. As a general rule, seeking advice of F1 colleagues is good practice, however only if there is potential benefit for the person in question. If sharing the problem with your colleagues will only result in further team disharmony or rumours being spread this is not a good response. Making an accusation about a colleague is not acceptable unless you have evidence. For example if the questions states that "you think" a colleague has behaved inappropriately this would not be enough grounds to be certain that your colleague is in the wrong and to report him to others as guilty. This does not however mean that your suspicions do not merit further investigation.

What You "Should" Do - It is an important but basic principle that the SJT questions are asking what a foundation doctor "should" do in a situation of ideal practice rather than what you "would" do. There are situations where these are differing. It is advisable to keep this in mind when answering questions. Publications such as Tomorrow's Doctors and Good Medical Practice give an invaluable insight and framework into how one "should" respond to given situations.

Preparing for the SJT

It is not possible to *revise* for the SJT, but it is possible to prepare as well as possible;
Attempt practice questions in books such as this, as well as taking the mock SJT exam provided online by the UKFPO online. It is usually best to take this mock exam under timed conditions to replicate exam conditions. It is advisable to do the mock 1-2 weeks prior to the real SJT exam. It is a good idea to go through the answers with some of your colleagues to gain a different perspective on the responses to a question.

Familiarise yourself with Good Medical Practice- The GMC's Good Medical Practice 2013 should be the basis of your responses to the questions. Following the basic tenants within it should help you to attain a good score in the examination. It is also useful to read the GMC publication "The Duties of a Doctor". Both are widely and freely available online.

Finally, and most importantly, experience in clinical practice as a medical student will be the most important help in answering the questions. The questions require a certain level of knowledge about how hospitals, wards, and the foundation programme function. This is best found on the ground during your clinical placement.

A nurse informs you that a diuretic that your registrar prescribed on the ward round is double the normal dose given to patients for heart failure. You have occasionally seen this drug prescribed at this dose but cannot think of an indication in this patient. You are not sure when the doctor will be back on the ward.

Rank the following actions in order (1 = Most appropriate, 5 = Least appropriate)

A   Tell the nurse to give the medication; the patient is stable and you have seen this dose occasionally before.

B   Alter the drug chart to reflect the normal dose

C   Wait for the prescribing doctor to come back to the ward then ask her for her rationale

D   Bleep the registrar

E   Go through the patient's notes and the BNF when you have time to check if this dose is indicated for this patient.

Correct response - DCEBA

This question is intended to test the sometimes competing interests of patient safety and workforce harmony. As the GMC makes clear, patient safety is paramount. Bleeping the registrar would be safest for the patient as you would get an immediate answer (D). Options C and E would potentially solve the problem but would take longer. Halving the dose would probably be safe but would potentially result in the patient receiving a sub-optimal dose and may threaten your working relationship with your registrar if she did actually intend the larger dose (B). Giving the medication as prescribed would potentially compromise patient safety (A).

Having just arrived home from a medical on call shift you realise that you forgot to handover that you had requested a Troponin blood test for a patient. You do not expect it to be abnormal, but you realise that the result needs to be checked tonight. You try ringing the F1 taking over from you, to no avail.

Rank the following actions in order (1 = Most appropriate, 5 = Least appropriate)

A   Go into the hospital early the next day to check the result and act on the result if appropriate.

B   Ring one of the surgical F1's working in another part of the hospital to check the result for you

C   Go back into the hospital to check the Troponin

D   Ring the sister on the ward to pass on to the relevant F1 taking over from you your concerns

E   Contact the Medical SHO to inform them of the situation

Correct response - EDBCA

Contacting the medical SHO directly solves the problem directly and quickly (E). Ringing the nurse involves relying on someone else to pass the message on (D) and whilst ringing another F1 is probably the most tempting answer the F1 will not have responsibility for your patient and your action in handing over the task to him would be difficult to defend if anything went wrong in the patient's care. The GMC states that your wellbeing outside of the hospital and home life is important (C), although even going back into the hospital comes above leaving the result until the morning (A) which seriously compromises patient safety.

You are an F1 on a busy surgical firm. Your shift finished 10 minutes ago, and you are leaving the hospital. As you are leaving the mess, your pager goes off.

Rank the following actions in order (1 = Most appropriate, 5 = Least appropriate)

A   Respond to the pager and carry out the task regardless of its nature, as you are still in the hospital

B   Answer the pager, note down the details of the job to hand over to the on-call team.

C   Do not respond, your shift ended 10 minutes ago, and you have already handed over.

D   Assess the nature of the call, and ask the caller to contact the on-call team if it is not vital that the task is done by yourself

E   Carry out the task if it is not too difficult.

Correct response - DBAEC

Reasoning; Although maintaining a healthy work-life balance is important, patient safety must always have priority (GMC Good practice 2013). Having answered the bleep (D), one can then assess the importance of the task; if necessary passing it on to the on-call team; if absolutely required for patient safety, carrying out the task yourself (D). Carrying out the task yourself (A,E) could damage your work-life balance, however ignoring the bleep would be difficult to defend (C).

The sister of one of your friends has been admitted to your hospital and is currently being cared for under a different medical team. You are asked by your anxious friend for an update as to her condition.

Rank the following actions in order (1 = Most appropriate, 5 = Least appropriate)

A   Refuse to provide any information

B   Explain that it would be against Hospital and Trust confidentiality policies to comply with his request

C   Liase with the team in charge of the patient's care, and ask if they will provide the required information to your friend.

D   Approach the patient and ask for her consent to read her notes and speak to her brother regarding her condition.

E   Get the patient's records and give the information your friend has requested.

Correct response - CDBAE

Reasoning; To avoid difficulties separating personal relationships from clinical judgement in the care of a patient, Good Medical Practice 2013 states that "wherever possible, you should avoid practicing medical care to anyone with whom you have a close personal relationship". Speaking to the relevant team (C) allows you to remain separate from the situation, allowing the doctors in charge of the patient's care to make the decision. Asking the patient for consent (D) is good practice but as she is not under your care and you have a relationship with her brother you should try and avoid getting involved with her care. Not doing anything at all would be rude and unnecessary (B, A) considering the other options available, but would be better than giving the information (E), which would be seen as a serious breach of GMC guidance with respect to confidentiality.

On the ward round your registrar decides that a patient under your care is ready for discharge. However, later on you go back on the ward, and the nurse asks you to reassess the patient. Having done this, you feel the patient is not ready to go home.

Rank the following actions in order (1 = Most appropriate, 5 = Least appropriate)

A   Discuss the patient with your consultant

B   Do not discharge the patient

C   Ask a different registrar for her opinion

D   Allow the patient to go home

E   Ask your registrar to assess the patient again

Correct response - EACBD

Reasoning; The key point here is ensuring that the patient is safe and well enough to be discharged. You have to be prepared to challenge a senior decision in the interests of patient safety (GMC Good Medical Practice, 2013). The patient's condition may have changed, so it is appropriate to ask the registrar, who knows the patient well, to reassess (E). Going above the registrars head and contacting the consultant (A) is not best practice but better than the other options. Asking another registrar to see the patient (C) would most probably maintain patient safety, but may cause problems between yourself and your registrar. Allowing the patient to go home in the belief that she is not well enough is the worst option (D).

Robert, a 20 year old with Crohn's disease has presented to A&E with a flare of his symptoms. You have told Robert and his family that he will be having a CT scan within the next couple of hours. However, when you discuss the scan with radiology they advise that they will not be able to fit Robert's scan in until tomorrow afternoon.

Rank the following actions in order (1 = Most appropriate, 5 = Least appropriate)

A   Refer Robert and his family to PALS and provide a leaflet on hospital complaints procedure

B   Explain politely that emergency scans must take priority

C   Tell Robert that this is the fault of the Radiology department

D   Tell Robert that you were acting on the information that you had at the time

E   Apologise to Robert and ask if there is anything else you can do to help whilst listening to his concerns

Correct response – EBDAC

This question examines your ability to diffuse a potentially difficult situation. Passing the blame for what you have said onto your colleagues is obviously inappropriate and will not promote team working or indeed help the patient himself (C). Listening to Robert and his family and attempting to allay his concerns is the best response (E). Patients and their families will often understand that emergency scans must take priority and accept this as an explanation(B). Escalating the situation by advising the family about the possibility of a formal complaint procedure would be an overreaction to the situation unless Robert is still distressed by the situation after you have attempted to allay their concerns (A).

You are a foundation doctor working in a busy medical admissions unit. Your shift is due to finish at 7pm and you have arranged to see friends for a meal afterwards. However your F1 colleague taking over from you rings to say that unfortunately they are running late and will not be there until 7.30pm.

Rank the following actions in order (1 = Most appropriate, 5 = Least appropriate)

A   Write a handover and stick it up on the ward noticeboard in the corridor where your colleague will see it

B   Write a handover in all of the patient's notes

C   Handover to the SHO if they are not too busy and ask them to do the same to your F1 colleague when he arrives

D   Leave at 7pm without handing over

E   Wait until your colleague arrives to handover in person

Correct response - CEBAD

This question covers handover, a vital part of looking after patients. Additionally it brings in aspects of work-life balance, which is an important part of being a foundation doctor. However, as always patient safety must come first. Patient confidentiality is also involved in this question. There is not perfect answer, but if your immediate senior is not too busy then it would maintain patient safety to handover to him (although you are relying on him to handover to the F1). This option would also allow you to leave on time (C).Waiting for your colleague to arrive is the next best option as this maintains patient safety although there is no guarantee when your colleague will arrive, so this could badly delay you. Writing in the notes (B) may seem a good idea but is time consuming and there is no guarantee that your colleague will look in the notes so an effective handover will probably not take place- your colleague will not know which patients require his immediate attention. Leaving instructions on the noticeboard will probably secure an effective handover but is an unacceptable breach of patient confidentiality (A). Leaving without handing-over potentially risks patient safety (D).

Your SpR has asked you to prescribe a medication for a patient, Mr Lovell. You are aware that Mr Lovell is allergic to a similar medication and are worried that a reaction may occur if you prescribe this medication.

Rank the following actions in order (1 = Most appropriate, 5 = Least appropriate)

A   Prescribe the medication and ask the nurse to observe for any reaction

B   Relay your concerns to the nurse

C   Ring pharmacy to ask their advice

D   Explain to the SpR your concerns

E   Speak to your consultant and ask their advice

Correct response - DCBEA

This question examines your ability to protect patient safety. A basic principle is that if you are concerned about prescribing a medication, you should seek further advice, even if you are simply following instructions (A). As the prescribing doctor (with your signature on the drug chart) the prescription and any reaction to the medication would be your responsibility, even if the SpR had asked you to prescribe it. The best course of action would be to politely query the medication with the relevant SpR (D). Pharmacy will be a good source of independent and expert advice (C). Speaking to the nurse would be good practice because they will be the person to give the medication, so will also have some responsibility and therefore would need to know about your concerns (B). Your consultant may be difficult to get hold of and this is not as good as speaking to the SpR concerned (E).

You are a foundation doctor working on a busy surgical firm. Over the past few weeks it has come to your attention that your F1 colleague on the firm, Alex is often handing over a lot of tasks at the end of her shift. This is despite the fact that she is often to be found in the mess when you feel she should be on the ward.

Rank the following actions in order (1 = Most appropriate, 5 = Least appropriate)

A- Approach Alex politely and ask her if there is any reason why she is often off the ward

B- Speak to the hospital's foundation programme director about Alex at the end of the year

C- Discuss the issue with your consultant or registrar

D- Try your best to complete the Alex's jobs that are remaining at the end of the shift to try and lessen the number Alex hands over

E- Discuss the situation with one of your F1 colleagues

Correct response - ACEDB

This question is designed to assess your ability to deal with workplace issues that will inevitably arise. These are far from unique to medicine. The important consideration in this case is whether you feel patient care is being compromised- this may not be the case since the jobs are being handed over. A further important consideration is the welfare of you colleague- there may be a legitimate reason why Alex is struggling. Therefore, giving Alex a chance to give an explanation is the first response (A). Speaking to a senior will provide an objective opinion and they will then be able to take the matter further for you if they feel necessary (C). Discussing with one of your colleagues is usually a good idea if you need some advice about how to proceed (E). Option D will compromise your work-life balance and ultimately not solve the problem or help Alex in the longer term. Option B would also not solve the problem until the end of the F1 year, and this is escalating the situation before giving Alex the chance to explain the situation or attempt to alter her practice.

You are an F1 covering the wards on a busy Sunday. Your colleague informs you that your F2, Sam, has called in sick this morning, and a locum has been found to replace him. You are aware that Sam was out with friends last night in a nightclub.

Rank the following actions in order (1 = Most appropriate, 5 = Least appropriate)

A- Carry out the job as normal

B- Inform the relevant consultant that you do not believe Sam is genuinely ill

C- Ring Sam and find out how he is, politely ask for an explanation

D- Ask another Foundation doctor for advice

E- Inform the programme director at the end of the year that Sam did not perform his duty as he should have

Correct response - CDABE

This question covers aspects of patient safety as well as your ability to work in a professional fashion. The best response would be to contact Sam directly to get an explanation- despite the hints in the question he may be genuinely ill (C). Asking a fellow colleague for advice in this situation is usually good practice, and to be recommended before escalating further. Options B and E are ranked below A because if you have no evidence that Sam is not genuinely ill then it would be inappropriate to cast aspersions about Sam to the consultant or foundation director before he has had adequate opportunity to explain himself- especially as in this case patient safety does not appear to be compromised as a locum has been found.

You are an F1 working in Orthopaedics. An elderly, frail gentleman who has had a fractured neck of femur is being discharged home today, and his wife has arrived to help him get home. His discharge medications will not be ready for at least 3 hours, but his wife has told you that she cannot wait that long.

Rank the following actions in order (1 = Most appropriate, 5 = Least appropriate)

A- Tell the wife she needs to wait

B- Contact Pharmacy and explain the situation

C- Allow the patient to go home, on the proviso that his wife picks up the relevant medications tomorrow

D- Apologise to the wife and explain that Pharmacy is very busy

E- Advise the wife she can come back tomorrow to take her husband home

Correct response - BDAEC

Ringing Pharmacy and explaining the problem is the only response that will potentially solve the situation in a timely fashion that will please all parties. They may be able to expedite the preparation of his medications. Explaining politely the situation to the wife (D) is better than being blunt (A), and may be more conducive to her co-operation. Keeping the patient in overnight (E) maintains patient safety but is inappropriate as the patient is medically fit for discharge and keeping him in hospital for this reason would be inconvenient for all parties. It is vital in this situation that the patient does not leave the hospital without his medication, therefore option C is ranked bottom- the patient will not receive any medications that he needs for the evening and there is no guarantee that the wife will pick up the medications tomorrow. This option is the only one that compromises patient safety so is ranked least appropriate.

You are working an on-call shift in surgery. You are asked by a nurse to prescribe prophylactic antibiotics for a patient that is having an elective gall bladder removal tomorrow. Having checked the patient's allergy status you should –

Rank the following actions in order (1 = Most appropriate, 5 = Least appropriate)

A   Check the local guidelines as to which antibiotic to prescribe

B   Check the BNF

C   Prescribe what you think is the correct antibiotic

D   Ask the on call registrar who is on the ward

E   Ask the nurse what to prescribe

Correct response - DABCE

This is a common dilemma during on call shifts. The safest and quickest response would be to simply ask your registrar (D). Hospitals often have good local guidelines as to what antibiotics surgeons prescribe prophylactically for each type of surgery (A) which may be different from what the BNF recommends (B). All of the above options would be safe. Prescribing based on your own knowledge if you are unsure (C) or a nurses recommendation (E) potentially risks patient safety. As you are the doctor signing the prescription you should not rely on someone else to tell you what to prescribe as it is your responsibility and it is not safe to do so.

A 45 year old lady who has been treated for breast cancer has been admitted with a spinal fracture. The radiological imaging is suggestive of metastatic disease to the bone having led to the fracture, however the images have not yet been reported. The patient says that she has a visit from her husband and young children later this afternoon, and asks if you think her fracture is caused by her cancer.

Rank the following actions in order (1 = Most appropriate, 5 = Least appropriate)

A   As there is no radiological report, tell her the fracture was not caused by the cancer

B   Ask a senior member of your team to review the imaging and discuss it with the patient

C   Tell the patient that her cancer has metastasised

D   Tell the patient you will discuss it when the results are available

E   Tell the patient that one of the potential causes is cancer, but the definitive cause is not yet known

Correct response - BEDCA

This question examines your ability to communicate with patients and also recognise the limits of your responsibility as an F1. There will often be a degree of uncertainty regarding a patient's diagnosis or treatment when you talk to them or their families, and this is to be expected. However it would not be responsible as an F1 for you to be telling a patient a diagnosis as important and life-changing as this without clinical evidence (in this case a radiological report) behind you. This may however be appropriate for more senior members of the multi-disciplinary team (B). Telling the patient what they may already suspect (E) may introduce more worry into the situation but is the next best response, as it is truthful. Completely ignoring the patient's question is rude (D), but better than giving false information (C,A) which displays a lack of probity.

You are an F1 on a Gastroenterology medical firm. One of your patients has just been reviewed by a consultant Rheumatologist as requested, and a plan has been written in the notes. Your Gastro SpR doesn't agree with the surgical management plan, and instructs you to ignore it.

Rank the following actions in order (1 = Most appropriate, 5 = Least appropriate)

A- Follow the Rheumatology plan
B- Follow your registrar's advice
C- Find out why your registrar disagrees with the advice
D- Speak to your consultant
E- Speak to the Rheumatology team to gain a further understanding of their plan

Correct response - CEDAB

This is an example of a difficult question, with several answers that are obviously incorrect. Other teams will often come to review your patients. As an Fı it will often be your job to read the notes and enact their plans. However it is not usually the job of an Fı to decide whether to follow senior advice- ignoring senior experienced advice is usually irresponsible and could harm patient safety. In this case the simplest solution would be to ask why the registrar disagrees with the plan-there may be a very good reason to not implement the plan (C). Speaking to a member of the rheumatology team about their plan may offer a further insight (E). If your registrar does not want to implement the plan, ultimately you should contact your consultant who is responsible overall for the patient. They are probably the only one who can make the final decision to ignore the consultant rheumatologist's plan (D). He may wish to discuss it further with his fellow consultant. Choosing between the two obviously incorrect options (A,B) is difficult but ultimately seniority would prevail.

Your shift finished half an hour ago and you are about to leave the ward when a nurse asks to show you some blood results for a patient with chest pain that the lab have rang to tell her about. Despite you asking her to bleep the on call doctors to inform them she shows you the results. You notice a very high potassium level.

Rank the following actions in order (1 = Most appropriate, 5 = Least appropriate)

A-   Mention the result tomorrow on the ward round
B-   Go and perform a full assessment of the patient, including ECG. Start the appropriate treatment as you see fit
C-   Bleep the on call F1 and ask them to come and review the patient now
D-   Tell the nurse to contact the on call F1
E-   Explain to the nurse in no uncertain terms that she is in the wrong

Correct response -BCDEA

This is a difficult question. Patient safety must come first and the nurse may be correct to be so urgent. A patient with a raised potassium and chest pain requires urgent assessment (B). Bleeping the F1 is a good option (C), but there is no guarantee they will come to see the patient in a timely fashion. Asking the nurse to contact the on call team introduces another layer of communication that is unnecessary and further risks the patient not being assessed in a timely fashion (D). Berating the nurse is not the correct course of action- she has acted reasonably in this situation and this will definitely not help your working relationship (E). However ignoring the situation could harm patient safety so would be the least appropriate option (A).

You are a Respiratory F1. A patient is due for a chest drain to be performed by your SHO Luke, but she informs you that she does not want to be treated by him.

Rank the following actions in order (1 = Most appropriate, 5 = Least appropriate)

A- Find out more about why the patient feels this way

B- Ignore the situation

C- Tell the Luke what has happened

D- Perform the procedure yourself if competent to do so

E- Stop Luke from doing the chest drain

Correct response - AECDB

Patients who have capacity have the right to make decisions regarding their treatment. This can include what treatments are performed, and within reason, who performs those treatments (as laid out by the GMC). Finding out more about the ideas and concerns of the patient is usually a valid first step in situations such as these, and could potentially offer an easy solution. It is crucial that Luke does not carry out the procedure unless this is resolved. Option E is preferable to option C simply because it is clearer in terms of the procedure not taking place. Performing the procedure yourself (D) is likely to be inappropriate because you do not know why the patient does not want Luke to do the procedure. As an F1 it is also likely it is not professional to do this procedure without informing Luke or asking more senior advice. Ignoring the situation risks potential battery occurring to the patient (B).

You are an F1 doctor on a Cardiology ward. It is your first day since qualifying from medical school. The partner of your patient comes in for a visit with their two young children. You are aware he has just driven to the hospital, and you think you can smell alcohol on his breath. What should you do first?

Rank the following actions in order (1 = Most appropriate, 5 = Least appropriate)

A-   Inform the sister on the ward of your concerns
B-   Confront the partner
C-   Ring social services
D-   Document your suspicions in the notes
E-   Fill in a clinical incident form

Correct response - ABCDE

This raises questions around child safety (safeguarding) as well as the safety of other users of the road and other patients on the ward. It also raises the importance of realising the limits of your experience. Immediately informing the ward sister of your suspicions about the partner would be a good first step; they will probably know best what to do next in a timely fashion (A). They will also have more experience in how to approach this type of situation than yourself (B). Confronting a potentially drunk patient could have significant risk to yourself. However this is better than ringing social services (C) because it is more likely to stop the partner driving whilst intoxicated. Whilst ringing social services would be appropriate later on, in this immediate situation there is not much they could do in the short term from the other end of a telephone. Writing in the notes (D) would also be good practice, but would not be your logical first step as there is no guarantee that anyone would read and act on your suspicions prior to the partner leaving the hospital. Filling in a clinical incident form would inappropriate as a first step, as it would again be too slow to help the matter (E). Additionally, it would be incorrect to fill in a clinical incident form without confirming your suspicions.

A 39 year old lady comes into A&E with nausea and abdominal pain. A battery of tests have been requested, but the only one which has come back is the pregnancy test, which is positive. Her husband rings into the nurses station to ask for some information.

Rank the following actions in order (1 = Most appropriate, 5 = Least appropriate)

A-   Tell her husband you do not know what is going on with his wife yet

B-   Tell her husband that she is stable and will be OK

C-   Ask the patient if she is agreeable to her husband being informed of what has happened so far

D-   Tell the husband to ring the patient's mobile phone

E-   Inform the husband that it is likely his wife is pregnant

Correct response - CDABE

This question tests your knowledge of patient confidentiality. Consent should be gained prior to informing relatives of the details of patient care (C). This is particularly pertinent in telephone conversations. Another way of ensuring patient confidentiality is not broken is to ask the husband to speak to the wife (D). However there is no guarantee that the wife is well enough to receive this call. Telling the husband you are not sure what is going on is not the perfect solution and may only worry him further; however this does not break confidentiality. Reassuring him (B) is inappropriate because the question does not give you enough information to be sure that she will not come to harm during this admission. Option E breaks confidentiality.

You are working on a busy Colorectal surgery firm. Your shift was supposed to end half an hour hour ago but you are still busy. A nurse approaches you and tells you that one of your patients, Mr Anderson needs overnight intravenous fluids to be prescribed. What should you do next?

Rank the following actions in order (1 = Most appropriate, 5 = Least appropriate)

A- Handover the job to the night team.

B- Ask the nurse why the patient needs fluids and about his fluid status

C- Ask your F2 if she can help you as she has finished all her jobs

D- Go and see the patient to perform an assessment of this fluid balance with a view to prescribing the fluids when you have finished your other jobs

E- Prescribe 1 litre of Hartmann's in a slow bag as per the nurse's recommendation.

Correct response - BCDAE

This question again tests your ability to weigh up concerns about patient safety and your own time management. Asking the nurse why she thinks the patient needs fluids and about his fluid balance is always a good first step; this will help you gauge the urgency of the request (B). If your immediate senior is free to do the job whilst you are still busy there is no harm in asking for their help (C). This would be better than you doing the job as you are still busy with other patients (D) so this may delay the decision. Handing over the job may seem a good idea, but there is no guarantee that the job will get done in a timely fashion (or at all)- they may be busy with emergency situations. Additionally the night team will not know the patient as well as you. Prescribing the fluid without seeing the patient potentially risks fluid overload (E).

It is coming towards the end of your shift, and your patients Gentamicin dose for the day remains undecided because the Gentamicin level result from the lab has not yet returned.

Rank the following actions in order (1 = Most appropriate, 5 = Least appropriate)

A- Prescribe the standard dose of Gentamicin to make sure the patient gets his antibiotics this evening

B- Call the lab and ask about the result

C- Bleep your SHO for advice

D- Document in the notes that the Gentamicin level needs to be checked and prescribed appropriately

E- Handover the job of checking the Gentamicin level and prescribing the antibiotics to the night team

Correct response - BECDA

Ringing the lab is the most likely of these options to resolve the situation (B). They may be able to inform you as to why the result is not yet back, and possibly give you a timeframe for when it will be. They may even be able to speed up the processing of the result or give you it over the phone. At the very least you will be able to confirm that they have received the sample and are processing it, which is an important piece of information. It would be appropriate to handover the job to the night team (E), especially if the result is not due to be back for significant period after your shift is due to finish. Good Medical Practice emphasises the importance of the work-life balance, and this would maintain patient safety. Asking your SHO for advice (C) is unlikely to help the situation as they would likely tell you to do one of the above options. However documenting in the notes (D) risks the patient not getting their Gentamicin, compromising patient safety. Prescribing the dose without having the Gentamicin level is an even greater risk to patient safety.

You have a few patients to review on a medical ward during a night shift. You have prioritised them in the order that you feel they need to be seen. Whilst she is waiting for you to get to her one of the patients who is a known drug user gets increasingly confused and agitated and hits one of the healthcare assistants (HCAs) in the face.

Rank the following actions in order (1 = Most appropriate, 5 = Least appropriate)

A- Go to the patient and try to placate her
B- Prescribe sedation for the patient
C- Call security
D- Make sure that the healthcare assistant is OK
E- Fill in an clinical incident form jointly with the HCA

Correct response - DACEB

It is vital to act professionally when dealing with patients, even if they have been violent or verbally abusive towards members of staff. It would be a good idea to initially perform a quick assessment to make sure that the HCA is not badly injured (D). Even if patients have been aggressive it is often worth attempting to calm them down (A)- sometimes just the reassurance of a few simple words and the knowledge that she will be seen to can be enough to calm a patient down. Simple things like a quiet, well light environment have been shown to be efficacious in settling confusion/ delirious patients. Calling security (C) is often a good idea once simple methods of placating a patient have been tried- this will help to ensure the patient's safety, as well as the safety of other patients and staff. However the very presence of security staff may inflame the situation. Filling in a clinical incident form is good practice (E) but is not an immediate consideration when the patient is still potentially confused, aggressive and ill at the present time. A doctor should not prescribe sedation (B) until the patient has been fully assessed and other options have been exhausted- it should be almost a last resort option. It can make the patient's medical condition significantly deteriorate depending on the underlying cause of the confusion/ aggression.

You are an FI working in A&E. An 18 year old girl, Kaliane, comes into the department heavily intoxicated after binge-drinking after an argument with her father about her partying lifestyle. She is now fit and well and fit for discharge. Kaliane's father comes in to visit her, but she has been asleep and so he comes to ask you about her condition.

Rank the following actions in order (1 = Most appropriate, 5 = Least appropriate)

A- Tell the father briefly about her admission, but do not mention the bingeing

B- Do not disclose anything to the father

C- Offer to go and ask Kaliane for consent to discuss her admission with her father

D- Ask the father to wait until Kaliane wakes up

E- Inform the father about her condition as he is her next of kin and she is only 18

Correct response - CDBAE

This question deals with patient confidentiality. Kaliane has the right to keep her details of her admission private, even though her father is her next of kin and she is only 18 years old. Asking for consent from the patient is the correct course of action (C,D). Not disclosing any details of Kaliane's admission may be distressing for the father (B) but is better than breaking confidentiality (A,E).

Your F2 colleague has a chest infection and asks you to prescribe him some antibiotics.

Rank the following actions in order (1 = Most appropriate, 5 = Least appropriate)

A- Tell your F2 to take some antibiotics from the ward drug cabinet

B- Take a full history from the F2 and prescribe appropriately

C- Advise your F2 to go to A&E

D- Advise your F2 to make an appointment with occupational health

E- Advise your F2 to visit his GP

Correct response - ECDBA

You should not prescribe for people that you work with or people you have a personal relationship with. Advising him to see his GP is the best option and would provide a resolution to the situation whilst keeping you clear from prescribing for him (E). Advising him to go to A&E (C) may seem extreme but is better than the remaining options and will allow your F2 to be properly assessed. Occupational health is not appropriate for a situation such as this and it is unlikely your F2 would be able to get the treatment required from this route of action (D). Although the GMC advises that you *shouldn't* prescribe the medication in this situation (B) this is still better than advising your F2 to commit theft (A).

You see one of the medical students coming out of a consultants' office having attempted to make a referral. She is clearly very upset and says the consultant was very rude to her and would like to make a complaint.

Rank the following actions in order (1 = Most appropriate, 5 = Least appropriate)

A-   Advise her to speak to the seniors in her team

B-   Tell her to complain to the medical student sub-dean about the incident

C-   Offer to speak to the consultant in question with the medical student

D-   Fill in a clinical incident form

E-   Ignore the situation

Correct response - CABDE

However daunting a prospect it may be, the best solution would offer to accompany the medical student to talk to the consultant in question and explain the situation to him. This would be the quickest and easiest option (C). Speaking to the seniors in her team (A) would also be a good plan before taking further action such as making a formal complaint (B). Filling in a clinical incident form at this stage would be inappropriate before hearing both sides of the story, and this sort of situation is not what a clinical incident form is designed for. Ignoring the situation is possibly the easiest option but would not offer a solution and may lead to further problems in the future or a long drawn out complaint procedure instead of a quick solution to the issue.

Your F1 colleague on the ward, Sophie has called in sick increasing your workload for the day. That evening you see Sophie working out in the gym.

Rank the following actions in order (1 = Most appropriate, 5 = Least appropriate)

A-   Confront your colleague in the doctors mess
B-   Ignore the situation
C-   Tell her educational supervisor and suggest they speak to him about it
D-   Take Sophie to one side and talk to him about the situation. If he cannot give an explanation then discuss it with her educational supervisor
E-   Discuss the situation with colleagues and if Sophie has done this previously then report her to her educational supervisor.

Correct response - DECAB

Initially it is most appropriate to talk to Sophie about the situation and explore her reasoning (D). This should be done in a private place to allow him to confide in you and not to embarrass her.

Doing nothing (B) is least appropriate as his actions could have led to patient harm and this should be prevented from happening again.

Discussing the situation discreetly with colleagues (E) explores the problem and assesses if the F1 commonly misses work, but does not allow her to explain himself. Letting the educational supervisor know without speaking to the F1 first (C) ensures action is taken but doesn't allow the F1 to explain themselves.

Confronting her in public (A) is not appropriate as it victimises the F1 and may affect her ability to work in the team in the future.

A bedbound female patient on the ward tells you that she thinks her ring has gone missing. She recalls placing it in her wash bag in her cabinet the night before. She thinks that a HCA stole it when he helped her put it away. What should you do?

Rank the following actions in order (1 = Most appropriate, 5 = Least appropriate)

A. Confront the HCA that she has accused
B. Inform the consultant looking after the patient and ask their advice on what action to take
C. With consent from the patient search her bedside for the ring
D. Phone the local police and inform them of the situation
E. Ask the nurse to complete an incident form

Correct response - BCEDA

The first point of call would be to consult your senior in the matter (B) as sifting through her belongings (C) could put you at risk and may lead to accusations against you. However this is the only way to establish if it has gone missing so is next appropriate. We should listen to all complaints, take them seriously, and complete an incident form if necessary (E). The local police are unlikely to investigate the matter but they can add it to their records in case there is a pattern of thefts (D). Avoid confronting the member of staff initially as the complaint hasn't been explored and it could cause un-necessary tension in the work place (A).

During a night shift you walk into the treatment room and find your SHO Michele drinking from a hip flask, and there is a faint smell of alcohol. She immediately hides the flask and looks embarrassed. She does not appear drunk. What action should you take?

Rank the following actions in order (1 = Most appropriate, 5 = Least appropriate)

A- Immediately confront her about what you have witnessed, stop her working, and report her to her educational supervisor

B- Ignore your suspicions and continue with your shift as she doesn't appear drunk.

C- Discuss the situation with her. Don't stop her working as she doesn't appear drunk and it would be hard to get staff to cover.

D- Discuss the situation with her and offer to help her. Organise for someone to cover her shift

E- Organise for someone to cover her shift and discuss the events with the team in the morning.

Correct response- DAECB

It is important that she does not continue working following alcohol intake whilst maintaining care for the patients by organising a locum (D). Option A leads to the same outcome but is less supportive to your colleague.

Waiting until the next morning is less suitable and the SHO's confidentiality is being breached by telling other team members about the incident, probably affect her ability to work in the team in future.

Allowing the SHO to continue working is not acceptable (C,B) which could compromise patient safety. Ignoring the incident (B) is the worst option as you do not acknowledge how serious the incident is.

You are an FY1 in general surgery. One of your friends who works for a theatre production company has asked you if you can get hold of some surgical gowns and masks from the operating theatre's supplies.

Rank the following actions in order (1 = Most appropriate, 5 = Least appropriate)

A   Refuse and explain to your friend that he will have to buy the equipment through the appropriate channels.

B   Take the equipment without telling anyone

C   Ask the person in charge of stocking theatres if you can take the equipment

D   Report your friend to the police for asking you to steal equipment

E   Refuse but give your friend the contact details of the person in charge of stocking theatres so they can find out how to get the equipment.

Correct response – AECBD

The most appropriate answer in this scenario is A as all of the other options have some degree of either dishonesty or unprofessionalism. The least appropriate options are B and D. D is ranked lower as it is a completely inappropriate use of police time although B is also a poor choice as it shows a lack of honesty and integrity. When deciding between options C and E option E is slightly worse as it may put them in an uncomfortable position and will waste their time as opposed to asking them directly if you can take the equipment yourself. This option may well result in them giving you the appropriate information on where to source the equipment.

You are an FY1 in general medicine. You are in the side room where the SHO is attempting to cannulate a recently admitted unconscious patient with a suspected heroin overdose. Whilst cannulating the patient the SHO sustains a needlestick injury. The SHO has important exams next week and therefore is reluctant to see occupational health as they are concerned they will be started on antiretroviral drugs which will interfere with their revision.

Rank the following actions in order (1 = Most appropriate, 5 = Least appropriate)

A   Agree with the SHO that they should not tell anyone
B   Report the SHO to the GMC
C   Encourage the SHO to see occupational health
D   Report the SHO to occupational health
E   Take a blood sample from the unconscious patient to find out their communicable disease status

Correct answer - CDBEA

The most appropriate option here is to encourage the SHO to see occupational health and therefore follow the appropriate guidelines for needlestick injuries. The least appropriate option is A as this will potentially be both damaging to the SHO themselves and also any patients that they may treat in the future if there is a potential risk for transmission of blood borne viruses. E is the next least appropriate option as the patient is unable to consent to giving the sample and whilst it is likely that this will happen it is not your responsibility as an FYı to be taking this blood sample at this stage. Option B seems disproportionate at this stage when you have yet to escalate the problem within the hospital services and therefore option D is ranked above it.

You are an FY1 in general medicine. You realise after reading the notes that you have accidentally prescribed a course of amoxicillin to a penicillin allergic patient which has just been given by the nurse. The patient has previously had an anaphylactic reaction to penicillin.

Rank the following actions in order (1 = Most appropriate, 5 = Least appropriate)

A   Don't tell anyone and hope the patient does not develop a reaction

B   Report the nurse who administered the medication to the sister in charge on the ward

C   Immediately assess the patient for possible signs of anaphylaxis

D   Cross the amoxicillin off the patient's drug chart

E   Inform the patient of the error you have made and apologise

Correct answer - CEDBA

In this scenario there are two clearly wrong options and three sensible options. Of the least appropriate options A is the worst as it would mean no action is taken and the issue may not be raised again leaving the patient susceptible to further harm. B is not an appropriate option as although the nurse should take some responsibility for administering the drug, it is the responsibility of the prescriber to ensure it is safe to give a particular medication. Option C is the most appropriate initial option as it will ensure the patient's health does not suffer due to the initial dose of amoxicillin. Option E is more appropriate than option D as the GMC state in Good Medical Practice that you must apologise to patients if you have made a mistake. Option D is also an appropriate response however this fails to take responsibility for the mistake that has been made and it is the patient's right to know this.

You are an FYI on a busy orthopaedic firm. One of your FYI colleagues has recently left the trust and has not been replaced. You have subsequently found your workload has increased to a point where you feel patient safety may be compromised.

Rank the following actions in order (1 = Most appropriate, 5 = Least appropriate)

A   Discuss the situation with you clinical supervisor that you feel you need more support
B   Write a letter to the HR department demanding that a new FYI is appointed
C   Refuse to stay beyond your contracted hours in order to cover the increased workload
D   Ask a fellow FYI on a different firm to help with your jobs
E   Record a clinical incident form

Correct answer - AEBDC

The most appropriate option in this scenario is to discuss the situation with your consultant as they will likely be able to make appropriate arrangements if patient safety is potentially at risk. If this option fails then it may be appropriate to record a clinical incident form if patient safety is compromised. This will mean that the situation is investigated appropriately and necessary action is taken. The least appropriate options are C and D. Option C would further compromise patient safety as no one will be covering these jobs whilst option D is also inappropriate as fellow FY1 colleagues will have their own patients to look after. Option B is not an appropriate option as this is not the appropriate method of escalation of this concern.

You are an FYI in endocrinology surgery. Upon entering the clinical room on the ward you think you see your SHO putting vials of medication from the unlocked controlled drugs cupboard into his bag.

Rank the following actions in order (1 = Most appropriate, 5 = Least appropriate)

A   Confront the SHO about what you have seen
B   Immediately leave the room
C   Discuss the case with your registrar
D   Report the SHO to the GMC
E   Discuss the case with your fellow FYI colleagues

Correct answer - ACEDB

The most appropriate option here is option A as the scenario states you only think you see the SHO behaving inappropriately. You will need to confirm this before any escalation through the appropriate channels. The next best option would be to discuss the case with one of your seniors preferably on the same team as you as they will also know the SHO and will likely know if there is any cause for concern. Discussing the case with your fellow FYIs may also be appropriate to get further advice. However, this could constitute gossiping and ultimately the case will need to be discussed with senior colleagues if proven right. The least appropriate option is to do nothing whilst reporting the SHO to the GMC seems premature at this stage especially prior to confirming your suspicions.

You are an FY1 in healthcare of the elderly. One of the patient's sons whose mother you have been looking after for some time asks to speak to you privately whilst you are taking blood. He takes you to one side and hands you an envelope which he says contains £100 whilst asking you to look after his mother well.

Rank the following actions in order (1 = Most appropriate, 5 = Least appropriate)

A   Refuse the envelope and explain to the patient's son that gifts are inappropriate from patients

B   Refuse the envelope and explain to the patient his mother will be cared for to the best of your abilities without the need for gifts

C   Accept the envelope and write a thankyou letter to the patient's family

D   Report the patient's son to the police for attempted bribery

E   Refuse the envelope and suggest the patient donates the money to the hospital charity

Correct answer - BEACD

Good Medical Practice states that you must not accept gifts that may affect or be seen to affect the way you care for a patient. Therefore the most appropriate options here are to refuse the envelope with option B the best. Option B is the option that will cause the least embarrassment to the patient's son whilst dealing with the situation appropriately. Option E is appropriate as the money will not be seen to influence the care you are personally providing. Option C is less appropriate as it seems potentially rude and ungrateful. Option D is the least appropriate option as the patient's son's intentions are entirely innocent and reporting them to the police would be wholly inappropriate in this scenario. This leaves option C which goes against GMC guidelines however is more appropriate then reporting to the police.

You are an FY1 on a general surgical firm. One of the medical students attached to your firm asks you to sign their logbook to say you have observed them and that they are competent at phlebotomy. You have never seen them take blood although they tell you they have taken it many times in the past whilst on different placements.

Rank the following actions in order (1 = Most appropriate, 5 = Least appropriate)

A   Find a patient on the ward who needs a blood test and ask the medical student to take the sample whilst you observe them

B   Report the medical student to the consultant

C   Sign the medical students logbook

D   Ask the medical student to take a blood sample from a fellow medical student whilst you watch

E   Refuse to sign the logbook

Correct answer - ADEBC

This is a common scenario that is seen in everyday practice. Whilst you may trust the medical student to be competent at basic skills such as phlebotomy, if you are to deem them as competent it is your responsibility to ensure that they actually are. Therefore the best option here is option A as it will allow you to decide whether they should be signed off or need more practice. Option D is less appropriate as option A as there is no need to take a sample from a fellow medical student unlike a patient on the ward. Option E is an acceptable stance to take although as a doctor you have a duty to teach medical students and it will mean the medical student is more likely to ask another doctor to sign them off when they are not necessarily competent. Options B and C are the least appropriate responses. Option C shows a lack of integrity as you are signing something that you cannot be sure is true. Option B is slightly better although still a poor response as there is no need to escalate this to consultant level when the problem can be dealt with easily yourself by simply observing the student undertake the procedure.

You are an FYI on a respiratory medicine firm. One of your fellow FYI colleagues on the team asks if they can leave half an hour early in order to attend a friend's birthday party. Just as they are leaving the doctor's office on the ward you are bleeped to assess one of the patients who has a low blood pressure. You still have a number of other jobs that need completing.

Rank the following actions in order (1 = Most appropriate, 5 = Least appropriate)

A   Go and assess the patient yourself and stay late to complete the rest of the jobs

B   Ask your FYI colleague to assess the patient before they go

C   Assess the patient and handover any jobs you have remaining to the night FYI

D   Ignore the patient and continue with the jobs you have left

E   Ask your registrar to come to assess the patient

Correct answer - BACED

The best answer in this scenario is B as this will have the least impact on patient safety. If the firm is busy then your colleagues should stay for at least the hours they are contracted to work in order to complete all of the necessary jobs. Option A is the next most appropriate answer as this will not have too much of an impact on patient safety although it is not fair for you to be taking a disproportionate amount of the workload. Option C is also an appropriate option although it may be difficult to explain why you have so many jobs to handover to the night FY1 when your colleague has left early. Options E and D are the least appropriate. Option E would be inappropriate as you have yet to see the patient and make an assessment as to whether senior help is required. Option D would potentially leave the patient with no one to assess them and could seriously harm them.

You are an FY1 in orthopaedics. It is a Saturday morning and you are living in hospital accommodation on site. You have forgotten to switch your bleep off and it goes off. You are not supposed to be working this weekend.

Rank the following actions in order (1 = Most appropriate, 5 = Least appropriate)

A   Answer the bleep and berate the person calling you for calling on a day off

B   Answer the bleep and advise the person calling of the bleep for the weekend on call FY1

C   Ignore the bleep

D   Answer the bleep and perform the task you are asked to perform

E   Don't answer the bleep but call the FY1 on call and ask if everything is ok

Correct answer - BCEDA

This is a difficult situation to find yourself in and tests the ability to manage as well as prioritise a work life balance. The most appropriate option here would be to answer the bleep and redirect the caller to the appropriate FY1 covering your work over the weekend. Ignoring the bleep is also an appropriate option as if you were not living on site or had switched your bleep off you would not know you had been bleeped. Ignoring the bleep but phoning your FY1 colleague would not be of much help as it is unlikely that they will know what the situation is at this stage. Answering the bleep and performing the task would be inappropriate as you may not be able to see the task through to completion without having to stay in the hospital for some time to follow it up. You would also need to handover to the FY1 who is supposed to be covering over the weekend undertaking the job once. The least appropriate option is A as this is both unhelpful in the situation and will likely cause unnecessary distress to the person who has bleeped you.

You have noticed that the final year medical student attached to your firm has attracted a few comments from patients with respect to her dress code, which they believe is inappropriate.

Select the three most appropriate responses to this scenario

A   Speak to the Sub-dean about the student

B   Ask the other Fis what they think of your students standard of dress when you are next in the mess

C   Ask the other patients on the ward what they think of your students standard of dress

D   Ask you registrar to mention the patients comments to the student

E   Speak to the student about the issue

F   Ask the student administrator to send an e-mail to the medical student, reminding them of the hospital dress code.

H   Tell the student to get changed into appropriate clothing

Correct answer - DEF

This is potentially an important issue that could lead to a formal patient complaint, therefore must be taken seriously. Additionally, this is an issue which could affect the medical student throughout her career if she is indeed dressing inappropriately. However, escalating this issue before discussing with the student would be inappropriate (A,H), as would sharing confidential information in an informal environment such as the doctor's mess (B). Your registrar would be a good person to discuss this issue with the student and would have more experience in this field than yourself (D). The student administrator has the authority to email the student in this instance (F) and an informal chat with the student would also be appropriate if you felt comfortable (E).

You are on a surgical on-call over the weekend. You review a patient who has had a hemicolectomy two days previously. You prescribe strong analagesia for the patient, who is in pain. The nurse looking after the patient refuses to administer the medication to the patient, as she disagrees with your decision to prescribe the analgesia.

Select the three most appropriate responses to this scenario.

A   Arrange a private discussion meeting with the nurse

B   Insist on the medication being given

C   Perform a further assessment of the patient

D   Write an entry in the notes stating the nurse refused to administer the medication

E   Ask the nurse the reasons why she disagrees with your prescription

F   Cross the prescription off the drug chart, you don't know the patient as well as the nurse

G   Ask your senior colleague on call for her opinion

H   Tell the nurse that you will fill in a clinical incident form if she does not give the medication as prescribed.

Correct response - GCE

Reasoning; In this scenario the nurse may have more information regarding the patient's condition than yourself, therefore it is important to obtain the reasoning behind her reluctance to give the medication in a polite but expedient fashion. Insisting on the medication being given (B) is likely to compromise your future working relationship with the nurse and could have adverse effects for the patient depending on the nurses' reason for not wanting to give the medication. Arranging a private meeting is too slow a solution to the problem and may leave the patient in pain (A). Assessing the patient again (C) may provide the answer, and seeking senior advice is good in this situation (G). However, a definitive solution is most likely to be found by asking the nurse for her reasoning (E). Options D and F leave the patient in pain. Threatening to fill in a clinical incident form without knowing the nurses' reasoning will probably harm your future working relationship with this nurse and will not benefit the patient (H).

You are asked to prescribe insulin for a patient who has high blood sugars by a nurse. You look at the BM on the patient's chart and prescribe the corresponding required dose of insulin. The nurse then realises that she has mixed up the BM's for two of the patients on the ward and the patient has received a higher dose of insulin than required.

Select the three most appropriate responses to this scenario.

A   Start a dextrose infusion

B   Explain how serious the error is to the nurse

C   Fill out a clinical incident form with the nurse and ward sister

D   Re-check both patients BM's immediately and treat appropriately

E   Report the nurse to the Nursing and Midwifery Council

F   Report the nurse to the ward sister

G   Explain what has happened to both patients

H   Ask the Diabetic Specialist Nurse to review both patients

Correct answer - CDG

If an incident such as this occurs, it is vital to attempt to correct the situation first and foremost (to protect patient safety) (D). Starting a dextrose infusion straight away is inappropriate because you are acting without knowing the patient's BM- this could potentially compromise patient safety and even cause DKA (A). It is important to jointly fill out a clinical incident form in a situation such as this (C) and vital to inform the patients of what has occurred, difficult as this conversation may be (G). Reporting the nurse to the ward sister or the NMC (E, F) are escalating inappropriately at this stage and explaining the error to the nurse should be unnecessary and is likely to be patronising and not beneficial to your relationship with the nurse as she is likely to already appreciate the seriousness of the error (B).

A septic patient was prescribed antibiotics and fluids by your team the previous day, with clear documentation of the treatment plan in the notes and in the drug chart. The next day you discover that the patient has not received the required treatment. Having ensured that the patient immediately receives the prescribed medications, you should next:

Select the three most appropriate responses to this scenario.

A   Ask another nurse to take over care of the patient to ensure patient safety

B   Speak to your consultant about the incident

C   Confront the nurse

D   Report the incident at the morbidity and mortality monthly meeting

E   Inform the patient of the error and explain you will take steps to avoid similar mistakes in the future.

F   Call a formal meeting for all the ward staff to discuss the incident

G   Ask the nurse taking care of the patient if she was aware of the instructions in the notes

H   Write a reflective piece on how to improve communication between members of the multi-disciplinary team

Correct answer - BEG

Good communication is a vital part of patient care. Having insured that the patient is now receiving the correct treatment, the next immediate steps to take are to ask the nurse if they were aware of the treatment plan; if they were then why it was not enacted (G). As you do not have all the facts, it is important not to presume that the nurse is at fault or confront the nurse in an aggressive fashion (C). It is important to explain the situation to a senior member of the team as they are the clinicians who have ultimate responsibility for the patient's care and thus should have a right to be informed in scenarios such as this (B). Informing the patient of the error is crucial, as outlined in Good Medical Practice (E). Options D, F and H are all plausible responses but not immediately actions that are required in the first instance.

You have prescribed some antibiotics for a post-operative patient on your ward. However, the nurse does not want to give the medication as he does not think the patient requires it.

Select the three most appropriate responses to this scenario.

A Prescribe a different antibiotic
B Tell the nurse to give the medication as prescribed
C Give the prescribed antibiotic yourself
D Review the patient's requirement for an antibiotic with your seniors on the ward round
E Ask why the nurse doesn't want to give the medication
F Review the patient again
G Speak to your SpR to ask for advice
H Fill in a clinical incident form

Correct answer – EFG

The best thing to do would be to find out the reason why
    the nurse is reluctant to give the medication- his
    answer will most likely inform your decision making
    from then on (E). It is always useful to re-review the
    patient if a colleague disagrees with your management
    (F). Even if you feel that you still want to give the
    medication it is always useful to seek senior advice in
    this sort of situation (G). Waiting for the ward round
    does not solve the situation now (D), prescribing a
    different antibiotic does not get to the bottom of why
    the nurse does not want to give the initial antibiotic
    (A).

Bill is a patient on your ward who has been treated for a pneumonia. He is grateful for the care he has received, and attempts to give you £25 as he leaves the ward to go home even as you politely decline.

Select the three most appropriate responses to this scenario.

A Ask your Foundation Director what course of action to take

B Thank Bill for his offer and inform the ward staff of his gratitude

C Accept the money and donate it to charity that the hospital is fundraising for

D Suggest Bill donates the money to the ward

E Ask your SpR what course of action to take

F Tell Bill to keep his money

G Accept the money and buy biscuits for the ward with it

H Inform Bill of the fundraising for a local charity that the hospital is carrying out and ask if he would be willing to donate the money to this cause.

Correct response; B, D, H.

It would be inappropriate to directly accept the money, whatever your intention to do with the money (C, G). Telling Bill to keep his money (F) may offend Bill as you have already politely declined and is not necessary as it is perfectly acceptable for small amounts of money such as this to be donated to the ward (D), or if he is willing, for him to directly donate to a charity of his choice (H). Thanking Bill is polite and informing the rest of the multi-disciplinary team of his feelings could raise morale on the ward (B). Escalating the situation by asking for senior advice would be inappropriate as this is not an important clinical matter. Additionally you will not necessarily have time to consult senior advice on such a matter (A,E).

You work on a busy surgical ward with Charlotte, a fellow F1. Charlotte has previously told you she is really struggling with the work load as an F1. She has once again been unable to complete her tasks, and asks if you would be able to stay and help her finish the tasks. You have a dinner party to attend after work.

Select the three most appropriate responses to this scenario.

A- Complete the tasks with Charlotte

B- Ask Charlotte what in particular she is finding difficult about the job

C- Suggest to Charlotte she speaks to her clinical supervisor about her struggles

D- Speak to Charlotte's consultant

E- Spend some time the following day exploring how Charlotte can be more time efficient in her daily tasks with her

F- Request some of the tasks to be done by the on call F1's if appropriate, help Charlotte to complete the remainder

G- Ask other F1's colleagues for advice

H- Leave on time

Correct answer - BCF

This question assesses your ability to manage the competing interests of a colleague who is experiencing difficulties against your personal life. Patient safety must also always be at the back of your mind in this sort of situation- if Charlotte is really struggling is this affecting patient care? The best response would be to tackle the current situation by passing on any routine jobs onto the Fi's on the late shift, as well as doing any remaining acute/urgent tasks with Charlotte before leaving (F). In the longer term, Charlotte's clinical supervisor will be the best person for her to talk to regarding her struggles (C) and will be best placed to offer solutions for her rather than yourself (E). It would still be sensible to ask Charlotte the simple question as to what she thinks is causing her to struggle (B). Going directly to Charlotte's consultant without doing this is inappropriate (D). Leaving on time may harm patient safety if there are urgent tasks to do (H).

You are an F1 working on a respiratory firm. A patient is admitted unconscious via the Emergency Department (ED) with a Pulmonary Embolism. Unfortunately the prescription chart that the A&E SpR wrote up has been lost and the patient comes up to the ward with a new chart which has a treatment dose anticoagulation prescribed in the stat section by a different doctor. This has not yet been given. The patient's brother, Mark, is an intelligent gentleman who has been with him during the entirety of this admission.

Select the three most appropriate responses to this scenario.

A- Give prophylactic dose anti-coagulation as a temporary measure to treat the PE until the original drug chart has been found

B- Ask the ward nurse if the patient has already had the anti-coagulation

C- Give the anti-coagulation as prescribed

D- Bleep the A&E SpR to clarify the situation

E- Take the new chart and go down to ED to look for the original one

F- Ask Mark if his brother has had the anti-coagulation injection.

G- Stop the nurses administering the anti-coagulation until the other chart is located

H- Ring your consultant to explain the situation

Correct answer - DEG

Bleeping the SpR is the quickest and safest solution (D). Making attempts to try and find the chart would be a good idea (and taking the original chart with you prevents administration of the anticoagulation in the meantime) (E). Stopping the nurses administering the medication is the next safest option, preventing the risk of a major bleed caused by the patient potentially receiving double the recommended dose (G). Giving the patient a prophylactic dose (A) could still potentially cause overdose, therefore risking patient safety, as does giving the medication as prescribed (C). The ward nurse will not be aware of what happened to the patient in the ED so it would be unhelpful to ask her (B). Relying on patient's relatives in such a situation is not acceptable (F) and would not be a credible defence if the patient did come to harm from receiving double doses. Ringing the consultant (H) would not help in this situation; he will not know what happened to the patient in the ED and will probably not help you find the drug chart!

You feel that your F1 colleague Alice has been making quite a few mistakes when spelling drug names and working out the dosages of medications on the drug charts.

Select the three most appropriate responses to this scenario.

A- Ask Alice if she feels she is struggling with prescribing, and if so why

B- Offer to check all of Alice's prescriptions with her

C- Inform a senior doctor on the team of your concerns

D- Offer to Alice to correct all of the incorrect prescriptions you see

E- Inform the nurse and advise her to check Alice's prescriptions closely

F- Inform the ward pharmacist and advise him to check Alice's prescriptions closely

G- Report Alice to the Foundation director

H- Tell the other F1s about your concerns

Correct answer - ACF

Mistakes in prescribing can be very serious, so this matter is not to be taken lightly. Even so, it would be appropriate to try and find out if Alice feels there is any reason why she is making these mistakes (A). It also allows you to inform Alice of your concerns politely, without going behind her back to inform others of your concerns without Alice being aware. Because of the seriousness of your concern, it is appropriate to inform a more experienced doctor on your team (C). They are ultimately responsible for the patients so if you feel patient safety may be compromised it is important they are aware of your concerns. The ward pharmacist will be checking the prescriptions on the ward, so it would be a good idea to inform him of your concerns (F). This will aid patient safety. It is unlikely you will have time to check all of Alice's prescriptions with her (B). Attempting to correct any prescriptions that you see may seem a good idea but there may be many that you miss (D). It is not the nurses role to check every prescription that Alice makes and she would not have the resources to do so, so it would be inappropriate to ask for this (E). Reporting Alice to the Foundation director would not be necessary as the Foundation director would not be able to directly help the problem. This would be escalating the problem too far (G). Telling other Fı's about Alice's problems will not help Alice or patient safety (H).

You are working with Jamie, a fellow F1 on a busy Medical Admissions Unit. Unfortunately Jamie has arrived about 15 minutes late for work every day over the past week or so, leaving you on your own.

Select the three most appropriate responses to this scenario.

A- Report Jamie to the GMC as his beahaviour could affect patient safety

B- Report Jamie to the Foundation director as his behaviour could affect patient safety

C- Speak to Jamie's housemates to find out if there are any problems at home affecting Jamie

D- Cover for Jamie for now; It is only in the last few days that this has been happening

E- Ask the ward sister what her opinion of Jamie's standard of work is

F- Speak to your SpR about the problem

G- Speak to Jamie about the problem and ask if there is any reason why this has started happening

H- Tell Jamie he must start coming in on time from tomorrow morning as he is affecting patient safety by not being on time for work

Correct answer - DFG

As always in this type of question it is a good idea to speak to your colleague to find out whether anything has been going on to explain his behaviour (G). Speaking to your registrar (F) is also a good idea as it is possible that patient care is being affected, even though he is only delayed by 15 minutes. If patient safety could potentially be compromised it is important to inform a senior. The only other appropriate response remaining would be to cover for Jamie for now (D). It is acceptable for you to cover for a colleague who is a few minutes late as long as this is not going on for a prolonged period of time- this is a courtesy which you would hope to be extended to you if for any reason you were slightly late for work in the future. Reporting Jamie to the GMC or the Foundation director (A,B) would be escalating the situation too far. Speaking to Jamie's housemates may be a breach of his confidentiality and may harm your future working relationship (C). Asking the nurses about Jamie's ability on the job will not help solve the problem (E). Being blunt towards Jamie without knowing if there is any reason for his lateness is likely to damage your future working relationship (H).

You notice one of the female porters crying in the corridor. This is the third time you have seen this happen in the last week. She confides that she is distressed by some of the comments she has received from her colleagues about her work and she is now looking for a new job.

Select the three most appropriate responses to this scenario.

A- Encourage the porter to report her feelings to her manager

B- Encourage the porter to ignore the comments

C- Encourage the porter to look for a new job

D- Advise her to go and see her GP

E- Attempt politely to find out if there are any problems at home

F- Offer to write her a good reference of her performance

G- Advise her to find a supportive porter to help her until she finds a new job

H- Offer your emotional support in the future if this were to happen again

Correct answer - AEH

It is likely that you will encounter upset colleagues during your time working in hospital. The most constructive way forwards is to approach their direct senior (line-manager) who should be best placed to attempt to solve the problem (A). There may be something going on at home which is contributing to the porters' unhappiness so asking about this would be a reasonable response (E). Offering emotional support to distressed colleagues is a natural and kind thing to do (H). Asking her to ignore the comments (B) is unlikely to solve the problem. Her GP would not be best placed to help her solve what seems to be a workplace issue (D). Encouraging her to look for a new job and helping her by writing a reference will not help solve the greater issue that may lie in the team of porters which should be addressed (C,G).

You are bleeped from Pharmacy, and informed that they believe you have prescribed an inappropriately large dose of morphine by mistake for a patient to go home with.

Select the three most appropriate responses to this scenario.

A- Write a reflective piece for you e-portfolio
B- Ask Pharmacy to not issue the prescription until you have checked it
C- Ask the pharmacist to alter the prescription
D- Fill in a clinical incident form
E- Inform one of your seniors about the mistake
F- Inform the pharmacist the prescription is correct
G- Inform the patient of the error
H- Write in the notes

Correct answer - ABD

Checking the prescription yourself and changing it as appropriate is the best and safest option (B). It is always important to learn from mistakes and reflect on them (A). Filling in a clinical incident form is important after any incident that has the potential to affect patient safety, even if the harm has been avoided (D). Asking the Pharmacist to change the dose seems an easy solution but as it is your prescription you are responsible for it. You need to go and assess whether the prescription needs to be changed, there is no guarantee that the pharmacist will prescribe the correct dose (C). Informing your seniors would not be helpful to you or the patient, and as patient safety has not actually been compromised is probably not necessary (E). Telling the pharmacist that the prescription is correct without reviewing it is not safe (F). There is probably no need to inform the patient of the situation as the prescription has not actually been dispensed yet. Writing in the notes is not necessary in this situation- there is no guarantee that anyone will see the documentation or act on it (H).

You are on a busy on-call shift when you are asked to confirm a death of a patient not known to you on one of the wards. The nurse tells you that the family are very distressed and asks you to come and perform the task as quickly as possible. You have 3 sick patients to see on your list.

Select the three most appropriate responses to this scenario.

A- Ask the nursing staff to help you by going to see some of the patients

B- Go to confirm the death

C- Ask the nurse to speak to the family and offer any support she can

D- Ask your senior on call to go and confirm the death as you do not know the patient

E- Tell the nurse you will not be able to complete the job as you have not looked after the patient during this admission

F- Ask one of the other on call F1s if they will help you with your patients if they are not too busy

G- Prioritise the jobs in order of clinical importance with the confirmation of death waiting till the others are finished

H- Speak to the family on the phone to answer their questions

Correct answer – CFG

Unfortunately this is a situation that will arise during your time as a Foundation Doctor. You must prioritise those patients that you can help, therefore you must see the 3 sick patients before confirming the death (B, G). It would be a good idea to ask the nurse to go and see if she can speak to the family and attempt to relieve some of their distress in the meantime (C), so they are not left in this state until you arrive. If you are exceptionally busy it is good practice to ask a colleague to share the burden with you if they are not too busy themselves. This will help to finish the tasks in a timely fashion (F). Asking the nurses to see the sick patients would not be safe (A). It would not be appropriate to ask a senior to go and confirm the death; there is no reason why an F1 doctor cannot complete this task and they are likely to be busy elsewhere seeing other patients (D). Any doctor can confirm the death of a patient, whether or not they have been caring for them during this admission (E). Speaking to the family on the phone about a delicate situation such as this is not a good medium of conversation (H). Additionally you have not even confirmed the death yet and are unlikely to be able to answer their questions

You are an FY1 in anaesthetics. You are asked by the registrar to insert a central venous catheter into a patient on ITU who needs one urgently. You have never performed the procedure before although have seen it done a number of times. The registrar has to rush off to theatre and will be unable to supervise you.

Select the three most appropriate responses to this scenario.

A   Ask the SHO on the unit who is competent at the procedure to supervise you

B   Wait for the registrar to finish in theatre before performing the procedure

C   Attempt the procedure unsupervised

D   Look up how to perform the procedure in a textbook

E   Gather the equipment you will need to perform the procedure

F   Refuse to perform the procedure

G   Phone the consultant who is in theatres and ask them to supervise you

H   Ask one of the ITU nurses to supervise you

Correct answer - ADE

A common scenario as a junior doctor is being asked to undertake tasks that you may feel out of your depth or need further instruction to be able to perform. In this scenario no FY1 should be expected to insert a central line unsupervised. It is therefore completely appropriate to ask for senior help and this may come in the form of an experienced SHO who may be competent at the procedure and able to give you some instruction. Waiting for the registrar to finish what they are doing in theatre may delay the procedure unnecessarily thus putting patient safety at risk. Attempting any procedure that you are not confident at unsupervised at is wholly inappropriate. Looking up how to perform the procedure in a textbook is an appropriate response as it will at least refresh your memory of the technique before someone can supervise you. Likewise gathering the equipment you need will help speed up the process until someone more senior can supervise or insert the line themselves. Whilst refusing to perform the procedure unsupervised would be in the best interests of patient safety this is less helpful than some of the other answers as the problem is not being dealt with. An SHO on the ITU unit is a more appropriate person to ask to supervise you than having to phone your consultant who may be busy elsewhere and although ITU nurses may have lots of experience in assisting in putting central lines in a doctor is a more appropriate person to supervise.

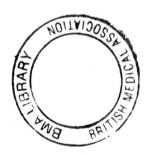

CPSIA information can be obtained
at www.ICGtesting.com
Printed in the USA
LVOW04s1228101016
507660LV00002B/89/P